Essential Oils

A Beginner's Guide to Aromatherapy using Natural Recipes for Health

ISBN-13: 978-1973739609
ISBN-10: 1973739607

Get Our Newest Books For FREE!

We love writing about ways to improve your health.

If you want to receive a FREE COPY of any future books that we release, please sign up to our VIP list.

To show our appreciation, after confirming your subscription, you will be able to download the FREE BONUS report below.

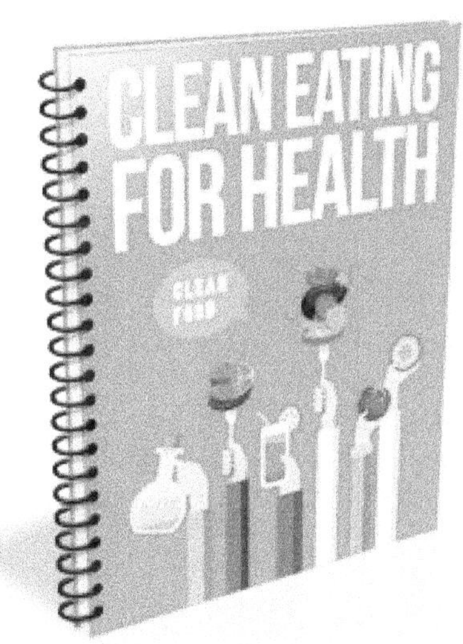

www.restrolla.com/VIP-CoBLo

Table of Contents

Introduction

Are you looking for an alternative treatment?

Do you want long-term effects without hurting your budget?

When it comes to an alternative, natural and affordable treatment, the first thing that comes into mind are essential oils. These are considered very effective for both major and minor health complications. You might need to wait a bit to see the improvements. But it will be more effective and will offer a lasting result. If you go with the immediate medical treatment, that might help to reduce the symptoms and to get an instant relief from the pain and discomfort, but these drugs will not address the root cause. The symptoms will be recurring. Moreover, these medications will affect the functioning of the other vital organs of your body if you take them for a long time.

You will not experience this problem with essential oils. These oils are fifty times stronger than herbs. Since they are oily, they pass through your skin straight into your cells and circulatory system. As the result, you can expect an effective result without any side effects.

There are many health benefits of essential oils. These oils can help you to have better sleep and to improve your mental health. Anyone struggling with depression can use essential oils to get peace and tranquility and to develop mental strength. Essential oils help to create a balance in your thoughts and to make well-planned decisions. You can use essential oils for the overall health benefits and cure some of minor and chronic diseases. As these oils do not offer any side effects, you can use them for people of any age. These oils can be used for a long time.

In most of the cases, you can also expect a rapid effect. These oils can play an important role in changing your mood and making decisions with a stable mind. You can use essential oils for stress relief, mood enhancement, balanced decisions, strong immunity, and for circulatory and respiratory health.

Essential oils are very powerful and effective. Even a small drop of an essential oil can offer you an expected result. Before using essential oils, you need to dilute them by using water, a carrier oil, or even vodka. Two types of carrier oils are normally used by most users for dilution. These are jojoba oil and almond oil.

You can use the essential oil for cooking, to get numerous health benefits. Essential oils can also be applied on your skin directly to improve skin conditions. For cooking, you need to use food grade essential oils. You should not use the perfume grade essential oils for cooking since they come with many added harmful toxins and can be detrimental to your health. Therefore, make sure that you are using only food grade essential oils for cooking. You can also go through the ingredients to know the benefits and potential usages.

You can use essential oils in different ways. You can use them in a diffuser to create a healing environment. There are three ways to diffuse essential oils. These are via a candle lamp, plug-in device, or an ultrasonic nebulizer.

You can massage the essential oil to create a stress-free environment and to get rid of the pressure of daily life. It will help to balance your mind and body. The massage will also help for relaxing your tense muscles and to get rid of a headache.

Essential oils can also be used in lotions and sprays. You can mix essential oils with the carrier oil and then use it as body spray. It will last throughout the day and will help to relax your mind and to remain active and energetic. In addition, essential oils can be used as perfumes, sprays, lotions, creams, and bathroom sprays.

Essential oils also work great for a toothache. They can help you with sore throats, toothache, and bad breath. You just need to make a blend of one drop of anise oil with two teaspoons of vinegar and then mix it properly. You can mix this blend with warm water and rinse your mouth with this water to get relief from a toothache and bad breath. You will get instant relief. You can continue this method for a couple of days for complete recovery.

You can also inhale essential oils to get immediate relief from a headache, sinus discomfort, stress, and sleeping disorders. You just need to put a few drops of essential oils on a handkerchief for inhalation. You can also add three to four drops of essential oils to a bowl of steaming water and breathe slowly to get the benefits.

Different types of essential oils are available. If you want to use these oils for health benefits, then first you will have to understand the benefits of each and every essential oil. You should know which essential oil will be more helpful for your digestive disorders and which one can improve your mental strength. A proper understanding of the usages of the different types of essential oils will help you to use the right one to get the maximum benefit.

You just need to blend different types of essential oils to get a synergy. The proper blend of essential oils can help you to improve your overall health condition. A proper blend means the respective power of each oil will help to enhance the other oil's energy and to achieve the synergy that you need to address a particular health complication.

A blend can be used in bath oils, shampoos, healing medications, body lotions, face oils, and shower gels. You can also use the blends for different types of health benefits. You can use essential oils for digestive problems, sleeping disorders, fever, joint and body pain, headache, cold, and for insect bites. These are affordable and will not cause any side effects.

Do you want to know more about the blends of the different types of essential oils? Are you looking for some effective remedies for your cold and cough? Do you want to improve digestive disorders with essentials oils? For all these, you can go through this *Beginner's Guide to Aromatherapy using Natural Recipes for Health* eBook. The eBook will offer you more than thirty essential oil blend recipes that you can consider using for different types of health benefits. All these recipes are effective and are included in this book after extensive research. These are proven, effective, and do not offer any side effects.

1. Essential Oils for Common Ailments

Essential oil comes with many health benefits. As mentioned earlier, you can use essential oil in different ways to cure both major and minor health complications. You can use essential oils to improve your digestion, to get relief from aches, to treat skin abnormalities, to improve blood circulation, and to cure breathing difficulties. If you have digestive disorders, you can use essential oils to get a lasting result. The best thing about essential oils is that they are safe and free from any side effect. You can use it effectively for any age group with the proper understanding of the blends. But if you use other medications, you might develop some health complications after a period of time.

Essential blend recipes for health benefits

1. For digestive disorders
This blend will not only help you to improve your digestion, it can also work as a great moisturizer for cracked skin. It is excellent for constipation, nightmares, and even for sleeping disorders. It can be used for children having nightmares and digestive issues. For this blend, you will need 9 drops of

orange oil, 6 drops of benzoin oil, 5 drops of Roman chamomile oil and 50 gm of moisturizer.

2. For joint pains

Anyone struggling with joint pain can use this blend to get immediate relief and a lasting result. It will not reduce the symptoms only; it will also address the root cause to offer long-term benefits. It will help you to get rid of the pain. It will warm and soothe your skin. For this blend, you will need 4 drops of yarrow oil, 6 drops of lavender oil, 2 drops of rose oil, 4 drops of Roman chamomile oil, and 50g of moisturizer.

3. For sinus issues

A sinus infection causes many health complications including a headache, nose congestion, and difficulty in breathing. This is an unpleasant condition. You will not find any effective treatment for a sinus infection. The process will be lengthy and the success rate is also not that satisfactory. But you can improve the condition significantly with the blends of essential oils.

Different types of essential oils are used to treat the sinus including tea tree oil, lavender oil, eucalyptus oil, menthol oil, sweet basil oil, oregano oil, lemon oil, rosemary oil, clove oil, peppermint oil, chamomile oil, thyme oil, pine oil, and geranium oil. To make a blend, you can use 4 drops of lavender oil, 3 drops of tea tree oil, and 3 drops of eucalyptus oil. You can place the diffuser close to your bed to get the maximum benefits. By doing so, you can inhale the blend properly.

4. For allergies

Most people have some allergies. If you have a weak immune system, you will be prone to allergies and a number of other diseases. You can use essential oils to boost your immunity and to fight against any kind of the allergy. You will find many helpful essential oils for allergies that include lavender oil, peppermint oil, lemon oil, Roman chamomile oil, and eucalyptus oil. If you are prone to cold allergies, you can make a blend of lemon oil, peppermint oil, and lavender oil with the same quantities. All these essential oils have anti-inflammatory properties. They can help you to get immediate relief from the cold.

While the lavender oil will help to cure a headache, peppermint oil and lemon oil will help to clear the airways by dissolving the excess nasal mucus. It can also help you to improve respiratory problems by clearing your nasal passage.

5. For cold and cough

For any cold symptom, you can use essential oil or a blend of essential oils to address the aching, fever, congestion, and inflammation. Lavender oil is considered best for colds because of its anti-inflammatory properties. It is also helpful to get relief from a sore throat and aching body. You can use the tea tree oil and peppermint oil for the congestion and to bring down fever. To prepare this blend, you will need the same quantities of the lavender oil, peppermint oil, and tea tree essential oil. If fever is a major concern, you can add a few drops of chamomile oil to the blend.

6. For Migraine

Migraine pain is really unbearable. Many people have this problem due to a stressful life. They use painkillers to get immediate relief. These painkillers might be effective for a time being, but it will not help you in the long run and the problem will keep reoccurring if you do not address the root cause. If you are looking for an effective result, you can use essential oils. Essential oils like the Roman chamomile oil, lavender oil, and sandalwood oil work exceptionally well for migraine pain. These essential oils can reduce the inflammation that causes pain. To make the blend, you will need 3 drops of Roman chamomile oil, 2 drops of sandalwood oil, and 3 drops of lavender oil. This blend can help you in severe migraine attacks. This is very effective for all types of the migraine attacks.

If you are having muscle pain due to the migraine attack, you can use a blend made with 2 drops of peppermint oil and 1 drop of eucalyptus oil. This blend will increase the blood flow to your brain and will also improve your cognitive performance. You need to inhale a lot of this blend. Therefore, make sure that it is placed near to your bed.

7. For motion sickness

If you are not comfortable with traveling and you experience vomiting, digestive disorders, and other complications during your travels, you should consider using essential oils to enjoy your journey and to make it more comfortable. For this blend, you will need 12 drops of fennel oil, 10 drops of ginger oil, 8 drops of orange oil, and 10 drops of peppermint oil. You just need to inhale this blend to prevent vomiting, nausea, and any other complication related to traveling.

8. For treating stretch marks

Many women get stretch marks during the pregnancy. They use different types of expensive products to get rid of the stretch marks. But none of them offer the desired result. Prevention is always better than the cure. If you prevent the appearance of the stretch marks, you will not have to be worried later about getting of them. You can use essential oils during the pregnancy to prevent the appearance of the stretch marks. For this blend, you will need 1 drop of Roman chamomile oil, 1 drop of lavender oil, 2 drops of frankincense oil, and 20ml calendula oil. You can also simply apply the calendula oil to prevent the stretch marks.

9. For muscle pain and itching

People with tense shoulders and a stiff neck can use an essential oil blend to ease the muscles. It will soothe the muscles and will also improve blood circulation. Moreover, it will help in reducing the inflammation and to get relief from the discomfort and pain. For this blend, you will need 1 drop of German chamomile oil, 2 drops of lavender oil, 2 drops of rosemary oil, 3 drops of marjoram oil, and 20ml grapeseed oil. Alternatively, you can use 3 drops of lavender oil, 3 drops of marjoram oil, 2 drops of lemon oil, and 50gm of moisturizer. All these essential oils are considered good for muscle pain.

Lavender oil also has the antiseptic properties that can help to heal cuts and insect bites. Lemon oil works well for the aching muscles and joint pains.

If you have developed itching and rashes then you can consider an essential oil blend made with 10 drops of Roman chamomile oil and 12 drops of lavender oil. You can use it as a lotion to get relief from the itching.

10. For fresh breath
If you have bad breath, you can use essential oil blends to improve the condition. For this, you will need a blend of 2 drops of peppermint oil, 1 drops of myrrh oil, and 1 drop of tea tree oil.

11. For sensuality
Essential oils are very popular for the fragrance alone. With the combination of jasmine oil, patchouli oil, neroli oil, geranium oil, rose oil, ylang-ylang oil, sandalwood oil, and clary sage oil, you can convert your simple bedroom into the most beautiful retreat. It will give you the feeling of being in a five-star hotel. To create your mood and to boost your confidence, you can make a blend of 5 drops of jasmine oil, 4 drops of ylang-ylang oil, and 5 drops of neroli oil.

2. Essential Oils for Mental Health

Life has become more stressful and complicated than ever. You cannot escape from the stress of day-to-day life. You need to build your mental strength to deal with complications with a positive attitude. Negative emotions, anxiety, stress, low mood, and failures will keep coming at every stage of your life. Instead of being a victim of these negative emotions, you will have to conquer them with your willpower and positive thinking. You can use essential oils as a mood enhancer. These blends can truly create a positive environment for you.

You will have many options in essential oils for your diffuser. You can use anything like jasmine oil, lemon oil, clary sage oil, bergamot oil, basil oil, frankincense oil, rose oil, geranium oil, sandalwood oil, wild orange oil, Roman chamomile oil, lavender oil, marjoram oil, and mandarin oil. You just need to use it in your diffuser to get the benefits.

While choosing essential oils for your mental health, you need to choose your preferred fragrance. You should never choose one that you dislike. If you do so, it will only offer adverse effects. You need to use the oil that will stimulate your positive emotions instead of using the one that will create negative ones. You need a tension-free, peaceful, and cheerful life.

Essential blend recipes for mental health

1. For a calm and stress-free life
If your job causes a lot of stress or your personal life is not that satisfactory, then you can use an essential oil blend to improve your mindset and to make it easy to be calm in all circumstances. For this blend, you will need 4 drops of sandalwood oil, 4 drops of ylang-ylang oil, and 2 drops of lemon oil. Sandalwood oil and ylang-ylang oil are considered effective for anxiety and the lemon oil can be used to enhance your mood. This blend can be used for any kind of anxiety and depression including personal and professional.

To create a healthy environment for your entire family, you can make a blend with the mandarin oil, rose oil, and jasmine oil. It will create a healthy and peaceful environment around your home.

2. For cognitive performance
People are considering different types of healthy drinks to improve the cognitive performance of their kids. They try these methods from an early age. Even college and university-students do research on how to improve their cognitive performance and to perform better. Many of them do not know that essential oils can be very helpful to improve cognitive performance. They can use lavender oil and peppermint oil for this purpose. Lavender oil is helpful in increasing memory and the peppermint oil will improve your cognitive performance as well. For this blend, you will have to make a blend of 5 drops of Lavender oil and 5 drops of peppermint oil. You can place this blend in your study room or office to get the benefits.

3. Essential Oils for Cleansing, Moisturizing & Toning

You need to use cleansers and toners on a daily basis to maintain your skin and to retain the original glow and freshness. You will find different types of cleansers in the current market. These cleansers and toners might offer you glowing and radiant skin, but the result will be temporary. Besides, it will damage your skin from the inside. If you choose the wrong product, you can have an adverse effect.

For those looking for a fragrance-free and natural cleaner, an essential oils blend will be an ideal option. These are cost-effective and can offer a lasting result. These blends will remove the trapped dirt and will cleanse the skin while soothing the inflamed area. Essential oil cleansers will serve all the basic purposes of a cleanser with some added benefits.

Some essential oils like bergamot oil, lavender oil, grapefruit oil, and geranium oil have strong antiseptic qualities that will heal your skin from the inside. If you are looking for anti-inflammatory properties, then you can consider something like chamomile oil or yarrow oil. For normal skin improvement, you will find many options including frankincense oil, sandalwood oil, cedarwood oil, benzoin oil, patchouli oil, rose oil, and rosewood oil. These essential oils are considered good for all of the skin types.

All these essential oils are also good for skin toning. For oily skin, you can use lemon oil, lemongrass oil, rosemary oil, and peppermint oil. With these essential oils, you can mix in the flower waters to get the maximum benefits. You can consider anything like rose water or orange blossom. You need to make a proper blend to get the benefits.

Essential oil blend recipes for the cleanser and toner

1. Citrus Cleanser

The citrus cleanser is good for all types of skin. It will help to balance out patches of oily and dry skin. To make this blend, you will have to use 4 drops of grapefruit oil, 2 drops of geranium oil, 50g of cleanser, and 3 drops of the cedarwood essential oil.

2. Cheer up cleanser

Cheer up cleanser will improve blood circulation and skin texture. It is also effective in improving skin color. For this blend, you will need 4 drops of rosewood oil, 3 drops of palmarosa oil, 3 drops of grapefruit oil, and 50g of cleanser.

3. Forest toner

Forest Toner is a soothing blend that calms and cools your skin. It is very useful to reduce the infection and inflammation related to acne. For this blend, you will need 7 drops of bergamot oil, 5 drops of sandalwood oil, 40ml of rose water, and 3 drops of lavender oil.

Moisturizer

Moisturizer is important if you want glowing, young, and flawless skin even in your old age. Without moisturizer, you cannot maintain your skin in the right way. Moisturizer can help to improve your skin condition and to reduce the fine lines and wrinkles. It will delay the signs of aging. If you are looking for a natural, fragrance-free, and lanolin-free moisturizer, you can use essential oils. Essential oils work incredibly well as a moisturizer.

Essential oil blend recipes for moisturizer

1. Orange tree
Orange tree moisturizer is considered good for dry skin. If you have very dry skin and find it difficult to maintain balance, you can consider using this moisturizer. To prepare this moisturizer, you will need 4 drops of orange oil, 10 drops of sandalwood oil, 4 drops of neroli oil, and 50gm of moisturizer.

2. After-sun
An after-sun moisturizer is very effective for sunburns. You can use it as sunscreen lotion as well. This moisturizer is also helpful for dry, uncomfortable, and scaly eczema patches. For this moisturizer, you will have to use 4 drops of yarrow oil, 4 drops of cedarwood oil, 8 drops of lavender oil, 3 drops of bergamot, oil, and 50 gm of moisturizer.

3. Sunscreen lotion
You can also make your sunscreen lotion with essential oils. This blend can work better than any expensive sunscreen lotion by protecting your skin from the ultra UV rays of the sun. To prepare this natural sunscreen lotion, you will need ½ cup of olive oil, ¼ cup of coconut oil, 2 tablespoons shea butter, ¼ cup beeswax pastilles, 1 teaspoon vitamin E oil, 2 tablespoon zinc oxide, 8 drops of lavender oil, 5 drops of helichrysum oil, and geranium essential oil. You just need to put all these above ingredients in a double boiler pan except the zinc oxide. Turn the heat to medium until the ingredients are melted. Then you can remove it from the heat and allow it to cool down a bit and then add the zinc oxide and mix

well. Now you can keep your homemade sunscreen lotion in
a jar for future use.

4. Essential Oils for Face, Hair, and Bathing

People use different types of cosmetics to improve their skin condition, to maintain their hair, and to meet their bathing needs. For all the above purposes, they spend huge amounts. But they do not get the expected result. When some products affect the density of the hair, others cause dry and unmanageable hair. The same is applicable to your bathing needs. People use different types of soaps to improve their skin color without knowing that these soaps are removing the oils from the skin and causing dryness. Your skin needs a certain amount of oil to remain waterproof. You need something to protect your skin from the dryness and to keep it young and refreshed for a long time.

You can use an essential oils blend to protect your skin from the damage that you normally experience with soap. A proper blend of essential oils can balance adolescent skin while clearing the impurities and leaving it supple and unblemished.

Essential oils can be used as body spray, skin cream, and body oil. You can also simply add the essential oil to your bath water. For the spray, you can make a combination of the 8 drops of the essential oil with 4 ounces of water. For the shampoo, you can use a blend of a few drops of cedarwood oil, lavender oil, and basil oil. For density or to increase the volume, you can add rosemary oil to this blend. To maintain your skin, you can massage a few drops of rose oil into your skin. It will improve the skin condition and will protect skin from aging. For the body oil, you can make a blend of jojoba oil, almond oil, borage seed, and sesame oil.

Essential oil blend recipes for skin

1. For skin clarity

If your skin color and overall appearance are affected by hormonal changes and you want to improve the clarity of your skin, you can use a blend of essential oils. This blend works well for teenagers. You can also use it in your thirties or forties. To prepare this blend, you will need 2 drops of lemon oil, 2 drops of sandalwood oil, 5 drops of lavender oil, and 25ml of jojoba oil.

2. Unblemished skin lotion

An unblemished skin lotion can help to get rid of scar tissue. It is also helpful for dry and cracked skin. It makes your skin become unblemished and supple. To prepare this lotion, you will need 3 drops of benzoin oil, 2 drops of frankincense oil, 2 drops of sandalwood oil, 1 drop of rose oil, and 20ml of calendula oil.

3. Anti-aging Lotion

People normally try different methods of delaying the signs of aging. They spend a huge amount for this purpose. But most of the products contain harmful ingredients and do not offer long-term benefits. You can use an essential oils blend to delay aging. This blend is considered best for wrinkled and dry skin. It makes your skin younger, flawless, and smooth. It smells heavenly and offers relaxation and sound sleep if you use it before the bed time. To make this blend, you will need 4 drops of frankincense oil, 2 drops of neroli oil, 2 drops of rose oil, and 20ml of avocado oil.

4. Acne cream
Acne is a common problem for teenagers. They normally use different types of creams to control the acne. These products do not offer any effective result. In fact, some of the products make the condition worse and leave scars for life. If you are experiencing acne on your face, you can use an essential oil blend to improve the condition. For this blend, you will need 2 drops of lavender oil, 5 drops of tea tree oil, and 1 drop of geranium essential oil.

Hair

Essential oils are excellent for your scalp and hair. You can use different types of blends to make your hair dense, to improve the blood circulation, to combat lice, to ease dandruff, and to make your hair shiny. The smells are also nice and create a positive and balanced environment around you. Essential oil blends can work for all types of hair. You can use these blends both as the shampoo and the conditioner. The essential oil blends will make your scalp healthy, nourish your hair, and will make it healthy and glowing.

Essential oil blend recipes for hair

1. For hair loss
If you are having hair loss, you will need a shampoo or product that can improve the blood circulation to your scalp leaving your hair refreshed and shiny. It will ultimately reduce the hair loss. For this blend, you will need 3 drops of grapefruit oil, 2 drops of lavender oil, 3 drops of peppermint oil, and 20ml of shampoo. You can use this blend as a shampoo.

2. For dandruff and flaky skin
This essential oil blend will help to improve the blood circulation to your hair. You can use this blend for overall

benefits including the treatment of dandruff and flaky, dry skin. To make this blend, you will have to use 5 drops of bergamot oil, 2 drops of rosemary oil, 3 drops of lavender oil, and 25ml of shampoo.

3. For hair density

This blend is prepared to improve both the quality and quantity of your hair. If you have fragile and thin hair, you can use this blend to improve your hair condition. Moreover, it will condition your hair with extra shine. For this blend, you will need 2 drops of sandalwood oil, 2 drops of bergamot oil, 2 drops of lavender oil, 2 drops of frankincense oil, and 20ml of shampoo.

4. For healthy hair

If you want to improve the overall health of your hair, you need to massage your scalp regularly with essential oils. Massage will improve the blood circulation to your scalp and will make your scalp healthy. For the massage, you can use different types of the essential oil blends. You can make a blend with a half cup of warm olive oil and 10 drops of lavender oil. Massage your scalp with this blend and then wrap a hot towel around your head for twenty minutes. You will feel relaxed, calm, and refreshed.

Bathing needs

When we think of bathing needs, a few things come to our mind including soap, gel, warm water, and soft music. People like to spend a few minutes in the hot tub to relax both the body and mind. If you add a few drops of essential oils to your bath tub, you will certainly feel better. It will enhance your mood and will prepare your mind for the day-long activities. You will feel refreshed, calm, and positive. You will be in a position to conquer the world.

For your bathing needs, you should use some essential oils that can make you feel lively and refreshed. You can use a blend of citrus oil and lavender oil. You just need to use a few drops of essential oils instead of using 10 to 11 drops. Two to three drops can serve your purpose. Essential oils are very powerful. Even a drop can do wonders for you.

Essential oil blend recipes for bathing needs

1. *Water sprite*

Water Sprite can help you to have a perfect bath in the winter morning. If you are looking for a bubble bath in the winter morning, you can use different types of the blends. For example, lemongrass oil can be used for muscle aches and pain, jasmine oil will regulate any hormonal imbalances, and coriander oil can boost your immune system. You just need to understand the demands of your body before using any of them. To make a blend, you can use 2 drops of jasmine oil, 3 drops of coriander oil, 3 drops of lemongrass oil, and 20ml of bubble bath. If you have sensitive skin, you can reduce the dosages of the jasmine oil and lemongrass oil. These two types might cause an uncomfortable reaction.

2. *Miracle worker*

If you want to build positive energy and a calm mind, you can use essential oil blends. Essential oils are considered very effective for your mental health. Frankincense oil makes you breathe calmly and neroli oil builds your mental strength. For a calm mind and clear head, you can use an essential oil blend with 4 drops of frankincense oil, 2 drops of ginger oil, 2 drops of neroli oil, and two drops of ginger oil, and 20ml of bubble bath.

3. *Zen*

Essential oils can be helpful to make your mind calm and stress-free. You can use essential oil blends for a clutter-free mind and for a beautiful smile. In addition, these blends can give you relief from muscular aches, chest pain, sinusitis, and it also strengthens your immunity. You can use this blend to protect yourself from the mosquitoes as well. For this blend, you will need 3 drops of coriander oil, 2 drops of vetiver oil, 2 drops of patchouli oil, 3 drops of palmarosa oil, and 30ml of the bubble bath.

4. Hand sanitizer

Essential oils can be used as hand sanitizer. It will also work as moisturizer and will protect your skin from dryness. For this blend, you will need 6 drops of clove oil, 4 drops of orange oil, 6 drops of rosemary oil, 6 drops of lemon oil, 4 tablespoons of aloe vera gel, 1 tablespoon of vitamin E oil, and 3 tablespoons of water. Mix all the ingredients well to prepare your homemade hand sanitizer.

5. Essential Oils for Sleep Disorders & Tranquility

In the current condition, we hardly get five to six hours of sleep. Even if these hours are dedicated to sleeping, most of people do not get enough sleep during this period. Their sleep gets interrupted due to the stress and many health complications. Some people find it hard to get three to four hours of quality sleep. Without adequate sleep, they do not feel energetic and active the next day. They take medications to improve their condition and to sleep better at night. These medications might improve the condition but they do not offer any lasting result. The side effects will be greater than the benefits. But if you use essential oils, you will certainly feel better.

Some essential oils including the Roman chamomile oil, valerian oil, lavender oil, bergamot oil, cedarwood oil, sandalwood oil, sweet marjoram oil, lemon oil, orange oil, clary sage oil, ylang-ylang oil are considered best for sleeping. Essential oils can be used for sleeping disorders and insomnia.

Essential oil recipes for sleeping disorders and tranquility

1. Quality sleep
The lavender essential oil brings your nervous system to a relaxed condition. The valerian essential oil is used to make you fall asleep fast. It also prolongs your sleeping. The cedarwood oil is used to minimize the automatic motor activity and it is also considered good to prolong your sleeping. To make a perfect blend for all types of the sleeping disorders, you can use a blend of lavender oil, cedarwood oil, and valerian oil. You will have to make the blend with 5 drops of lavender oil, 2 drops of cedarwood oil, and 3 drops of valerian oil. Anyone struggling with sleeping disorders can use this blend to fall asleep fast and to stay asleep for a long period. This blend will improve both the quality and the quantity of your sleep. Moreover, you will find yourself refreshed and rejuvenated every morning. If you are having nightmares, you can add a few drops of Roman chamomile oil to this blend to improve the condition.

2. Doze
If you are having difficulties falling asleep due to overwork, stress, and muscle pain, you can use this blend to relax your mind and to prepare your body for a sound sleep. It will make you sleep in no time. To prepare this blend, you will need 3 drops of vetiver oil, 4 drops of orange oil, 4 drops of lavender oil, and 30ml of grapeseed oil.

3. Tranquility
If you want quality sleep, you can add a few drops of this blend to your bathtub. A shower before going to bed will offer a better result. This blend will also help to get rid of exercise-related muscular pain. If you have dry skin, you can use this blend to improve your skin condition. To make this blend, you will need 3 drops of marjoram oil, 3 drops of yarrow oil, 2 drops of geranium oil, and 20ml of bubble bath.

6. Essential Oils for Insect Bite and Repellent Spray

An insect bite is very painful. In some cases, insect bites are dangerous. You can have discomfort, swelling, pain, and itching. You can use medications to improve the condition and to prevent the spreading of the infection. But you cannot use these medications without a prescription. The process will be lengthy and will make the condition worse. But you can use essential oil blends to reduce the symptoms and to prevent the spreading of the infection.

Essential oil blend recipes for insect bites

1. For an insect bite
You can use essential oil blends to reduce the symptoms of an insect bite. For this blend, you will need 10 drops of Roman chamomile oil, 5 drops of peppermint oil, 12 drops of lavender oil, and 6 drops of lemon oil.

2. Insect repellent spray
If you have a lot of insects in your garden and you find it difficult to control them, you can use essential oil blends to control their spreading and to prevent their appearance. This blend will not affect your plants. It will also spread a pleasant

aroma that you will not experience with the chemicals usually used to kill the insects in your garden. To prepare this blend, you will need 12 drops of rosemary oil, 10 drops of peppermint oil, 8 drops of clove oil, and 12 drops of thyme oil. All these essential oils are considered good to kill insects. But these are not harmful to humans. You can simply spray this blend on the soil to kill the insects or to prevent their appearance.

3. Bug repellent

Bugs are a common household problem. Many people have bugs in their home. They use different types of methods to get rid of the bugs permanently. But many of them do not offer a lasting solution. Even if they get relief for a temporary period, they do not get a permanent result. The bugs keep coming. If you are one of these people, you can consider using essential oils. This is an easy and simple method but offers an effective result. To make this blend, you will need 7 drops of lavender oil, 12 drops of lemongrass oil, 10 geranium oil, and 8 drops of peppermint oil.

4. For bacteria

If you want to kill the bacteria in your home and to make your living place more hygienic, you might need to spend a decent amount on chemicals every month. Moreover, these methods might not be healthy for your pet and your younger kids. If you are looking for a safe option and a lasting solution, you can use essential oils. For this blend, you will need 30 drops of clove oil, 25 drops of lemon oil, 5 drops of eucalyptus oil, 10 drops of cinnamon oil, and 3 drops of rosemary oil. You can use this blend to protect your home from bacteria and to kill them.

Essential oil blends offer different types of benefits. You can just simply take a drop of lavender oil on a cotton ball and can apply it on your skin directly to prevent mosquitoes. If you want to humidify your home, you can simply add 9 drops of tea tree oil. You can also use essential oils as a room freshener. You can use any of the essential oils of your preference. A few drops of oil will refresh the air and environment. Moreover, these are safe and will not cause any allergies. Even if you have breathing problems and you are allergic to the room freshener, you can use essential oils. These oils will not irritate you in any manner. You just need to choose the right essential oil and the blend to get the desired result.

Conclusion

Blending essential oils is an art. You need to be creative to make it fun and healthy. You can use essential oils for romance, heath complications, meditation, well-being, cleaning, for insects, and for a number of other things. You will need practice to develop a proper understanding of the blends and benefits. You might need some more research to figure out which combinations are better and can offer you more benefits.

Once you are familiar with the uses and benefits of the essential oil blends, you can use them for different types of health benefits. You can easily incorporate these blends into your daily life to live a healthy, relaxed, and peaceful life. You can use them anytime to enhance your mood and to create a positive environment around you.

To get all the above benefits, you will have to follow some precautions. First, you need to choose the best quality essential oils. Different types of essential oils are available with a wide price range. Some of them are genuine products, and other comes with fragrance oils. These oils might appear and smell like essential oils. But these are not the genuine products and they do not offer any benefit. In fact, they can have adverse effects.

If you want to buy pure therapeutic-grade essential oils, you will have to consider the best quality products. They might charge more, but these are worth spending on if you consider the overall benefits. Moreover, if you buy the low-quality products, it will not serve your purpose. The harmful chemical additives can worsen the condition instead of creating any improvement. If you feel that the essential oil blends are not working well and not offering the expected benefits, then you should inquire about the authenticity of the product. Besides, you should not buy old products. You should always consider buying the products that come with the same year manufacturing.

While making any of the above blends, you need to be careful about the quantity. Essential oils are very powerful. A few drops of essential oil can make a significant difference. If you do not follow the right quantity of the oils, then it might not offer the benefits. The effects will not be harmful. But it might cause some irritation and discomfort. Therefore, it is important to follow the measurements carefully while preparing the blends. In addition, you need to be extra careful while using the concentrated essential oils. You need to dilute them first and then you can prepare the blend.

You can use the blends for a long time. For future use, you will need proper storage. You should keep the blends in a cool and dry place. It is also important to keep the blends out of the reach of children. To avoid any confusion, it is always suggested to label the blends after preparation. You can simply keep the blend in a glass jar and label it. You can also keep the oils separately and can make the blend whenever required.

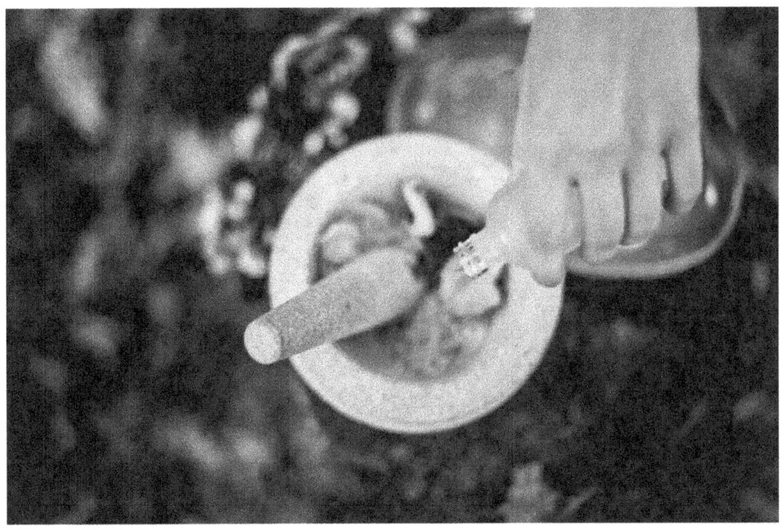

And finally, if you liked the book, I would like to ask you to do me the favor of leaving a review on Amazon.

Please go to your account on Amazon, or paste in the link below into your browser.

http://amzn.to/2uvjYKk

Thank you!

www.ingramcontent.com/pod-product-compliance
Lightning Source LLC
Chambersburg PA
CBHW050803240726
48654CB00008B/607